FIELD GUIDE ON RAPID NUTRITIONAL ASSESSMENT IN EMERGENCIES

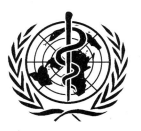

World Health Organization
Regional Office for the Eastern Mediterranean
1995

ISBN 92-9021-198-9

WHO Library Cataloguing in Publication Data

WHO. Regional Office for the Eastern Mediterranean

Field guide on rapid nutritional assessment in emergencies
/ by WHO Regional Office for the Eastern Mediterranean

vi, 63 p.-

1. Nutrition Assessment - Emergencies
2. Emergency Medical Services - Nutrition
I. Title

ISBN 92-9021-198-9   (NLM Classification: QU 145)

Designed by GRA/EMRO

Contents

Foreword

The Eastern Mediterranean Region has in recent years been affected by many emergencies, both natural and man-made. In almost all emergencies, nutrition is in danger, as people flee their homes, crops are destroyed, communication and transport become difficult, and the social structure of society is altered.

In the efforts to provide relief to those affected by emergencies, there is a need for data on numbers affected by, and on the extent of, a given emergency.

To estimate the need for increased food supplied, the nutritional status of the affected population is important information. Yet, those who are in charge often lack the know-how and expertise to give reliable information.

The WHO/EMRO Consultation on Rapid Nutritional Emergencies, held in Alexandria, Egypt, 19–23 January 1992, was called to develop a set of guidelines for the rapid assessment of nutritional status needed in emergencies, with clear instructions for use in the field, which would be compatible with the revised version of the WHO publication *The Management of Nutritional Emergencies in Large Populations*.

Experts from the Islamic Republic of Iran, Sudan, CDC Atlanta, FAO, UNHCR, UNICEF, SCF (UK) and WHO discussed and agreed on major problem areas in nutritional assessment such as choice of indicators, sampling requirements, methodology and analysis, use and users of the information. On the basis of this multi-agency collaborative effort, Dr Wolf Keller, WHO Consultant, and Dr Anna Verster, Regional Adviser on Nutrition, Food Security & Safety, wrote this field guide, with the generous assistance of Dr Ray Yip and Dr Kevin Sullivan (CDC Atlanta), Mr Robert Hagan (WHO Somalia) and Ms Rita Bhatia (UNHCR).

It is therefore my pleasure to present this *Field Guide for Rapid Nutritional Assessment in Emergencies*, which will guide the user through the entire process of designing, planning, implementing, and reporting reliable nutritional assessment.

I am sure that the *Field Guide* will be a useful companion for all those faced with disasters in the Eastern Mediterranean Region and outside.

Hussein A. Gezairy, M.D., F.R.C.S.
Regional Director, World Health Organization
Eastern Mediterranean Region

CHAPTER 1

Introduction

This field guide is intended for all those who are faced with the need to make rapid but reliable estimates of nutritional status in emergencies as a basis for subsequent action.

In an emergency, time is often limited and there is a need for immediate information on the severity and extent of nutritional problems.

As a result, data are often hastily collected and are later found to be of little use.

A group of experts from WHO, UNICEF, UNHCR, Centers for Disease Control (CDC) Atlanta, FAO, Save the Children Fund (SCF) UK, and representatives from countries of the Eastern Mediterranean Region met in Alexandria, Egypt, in January 1992, to review the minimum of information on nutritional status needed in an emergency for first decisions on nutritional relief and for its planning, and to develop a field guide for obtaining such information. The resulting set of standardized procedures is presented here. It has been written for use by the various agencies and to allow comparison of results from different surveys.

To facilitate the task of those in charge of obtaining information on nutritional status, the group made a number of decisions on issues such as minimum sample size, survey participants, and the level of analysis needed, striking a balance between the methodically appropriate and the logistically feasible. Decisions were based on scientifically sound methodologies and were meant to assist individuals with little statistical or epidemiological knowledge to carry out a survey that will yield reliable data for first assessment and for planning.

Those wishing to obtain more information on sample size selection, alternative methods of analysis, etc., should refer to the handbook on survey methodology published by the CDC, Atlanta, the UNHCR/MSF manual, or the WHO publication *The Management of Nutritional Emergencies in Large Populations* (revised edition). A list of material for further reading is given in Annex 8.

THE POSSIBLE OBJECTIVES OF A SURVEY OF NUTRITIONAL STATUS IN EMERGENCIES

- to diagnose the problem and determine its extent;
- to identify groups at highest risk, e.g. nomads, displaced groups, specific age groups;
- to estimate the numbers of people needing assistance;
- to act as a baseline to monitor the impact of interventions or the response to an improving or worsening situation.

In a rapid assessment of nutritional status in emergencies, the only indicator to be used is weight-for-height

The objective or purpose of a survey should be clearly determined before the start.

Those surveyed are usually preschool children.

In a rapid assessment of nutritional status in emergencies, the only indicator to be used is weight-for-height.

In addition, the presence or absence of oedema (see page 22) should be noted as oedema adds to a child's weight and so might confound the results.

CHAPTER 2
Planning the survey

Information on nutritional status will be of practical use only within the framework of the general situation in the country or region in which the emergency occurs. Existing knowledge on demography, mortality and morbidity, previous nutritional status, the socioeconomic situation, administrative structure, communications, etc., should be collected before embarking on a rapid assessment of nutritional status. This will permit an action-oriented selection of the study population and the planning of appropriate relief, which may not be limited to nutrition. Cooperation with other departments and ministries at an early stage is therefore essential.

Recent data on mortality are especially important for the interpretation of nutritional status and, if they are not available, they may be collected at the time of the nutrition survey.

The population to be assessed may be moving or living in camps, towns or villages, or dispersed in a rural environment. This will have important bearings on the design of the survey and the use of the results. Based on geographic information and available time, decisions will have to be made on the number and composition of survey teams. The type and number of trained, partially trained, or untrained personnel available will determine the amount of training needed, and the necessary equipment and transport. Such decisions depend in part on the sample design, which may in turn be constrained by the available resources.

The following checklist is meant to assist in the planning of a survey. Since this field guide is designed to help in making the necessary decisions, the relevant chapters are indicated against corresponding items.

CHECKLIST FOR PLANNING AND IMPLEMENTING A SURVEY

1. Which population is to be assessed (country, region, ethnic group, etc.)?

2. What is the smallest unit to be assessed (camp, village, district)?

3. Is there a need to analyse subgroups (by sex, age, ethnicity)?

4. Which sampling methods will be used (systematic, cluster)?
   See Chapter 4

5. Which age groups (6–59 months, 60–100 cm, 60–110 cm)?
   See Chapter 3

6. What will be the sample size? *See Chapter 4*

7. Which indicators will be used (weight-for-height, oedema)? *See Chapter 5*

8. What personnel, equipment, transport, number of teams, and resources will be needed? *See Annex 7*

9. Workload: how many children (clusters) per day per team?

Are the available resources sufficient to carry out the survey as planned so far? If not, review steps 1–9

10. Has a training schedule for field workers been prepared? *See Chapter 7*

11. Who will conduct the training? Where?

12. Who will supervise the teams during the survey?

13. Will data be analysed by hand and/or by computer? *See Chapter 8*

14. Are computers and operators available?

15. Who is responsible for the logistics (e.g. transport, equipment, accommodation, information for target population, etc.)?

16. Who is responsible for report writing and interpretation of findings (who is the target audience, what is the target date, etc.)? *See Chapter 9*

17. Who is responsible for taking action on the report's findings?

CHAPTER 3

Selection of survey subjects

In this simplified field assessment, nutritional status is usually measured only in children between the ages of 6 and 59 months. Frequently, children in this age group will be the first to show signs of undernutrition. They are generally highly vulnerable and in times of nutritional crisis may show increased morbidity and mortality. Children under 6 months of age (or about 60 to 65 cm long if age is not known), apart from being more difficult to measure, are often still breast-fed and therefore satisfactorily nourished. The upper limit of 59 months corresponds to approximately 100 to 110 cm in height of the reference population.

Because children in many developing countries are significantly stunted, a sample with the 110 cm cut-off will often include many children over 5 years of age and a correspondingly smaller proportion of the younger and most vulnerable children below 2 years. To maintain an adequate proportion of the younger children, it is recommended to use 100 cm as the cut-off point. At this stage, no distinction is made between sexes.

Target group for the survey: age 6 to 59 months or height 60 to 100 cm

In food emergencies, older children, pregnant and lactating women, the elderly, and the disabled may also be considered high-risk groups. They are generally not weighed and measured because there are no valid references for most of these groups. Since the status of young children reflects that of the general population, relief measures should also be extended to the other vulnerable groups if not to the general population.

It should be noted that, if many older children and adults are affected, the Body Mass Index (BMI = kg/m^2) can be used for an estimate in adults. The WHO expert committee on "Physical Status: the Use and Interpretation of Anthropometry" described the condition of low BMI as "thinness", with the following three grades:

Grade 1: BMI 17.0–18.49 (mild thinness)

Grade 2: BMI 16.0–16.99 (moderate thinness)

Grade 3: BMI <16 (severe thinness).

(WHO Technical Report Series, 1995, in press)

Selecting the sample

For a valid estimate, all children must have the same chance to be part of the sample

If an estimate of malnutrition is needed for a relatively small group of children, it is best to examine all of them. In a small population of, say, 2000–3000 people—of whom 18 to 20% may be children below 5 years of age (400–500)—all eligible children should be examined. In larger populations it is usually easier to examine and analyse only a sample of children and to draw conclusions on the probable proportion of malnourished children in the total population.

The first step is to define the population for which the estimate is needed. This study population is also called the sampling universe. The sampling universe may be the child population of one or several refugee camps, of a province, or of a country. The estimate will only be valid for the sampling universe as a whole. If separate estimates are needed for ethnic or geographic subgroups or other subdivisions of the sampling universe, each of them must be treated as a separate universe for which a separate sample must be constructed. Therefore, the smallest subdivision on which information is sought should be determined at the outset.

For emergency assessments several types of sampling are available:

No conclusion can be made about children who are not in the sampling universe

Simple random sampling: the children are chosen at random from a list of all eligible children in the sampling universe. This is the ideal procedure but usually not practicable in an emergency.

Systematic random sampling: children are selected systematically, say every 10th child, from a list of all households. Alternatively, if the average number of preschool children per household is known, a sample of households, say every 10th house or tent, may be taken systematically, and all eligible children in these houses are examined.

Cluster sampling: clusters or groups of households are selected from a list or from a map of all clusters; in each selected cluster a predetermined number of children is selected at random, systematically or sequentially.

Another approach to sampling is *stratified sampling*, which can be used with any of the above techniques. In stratified sampling the universe is stratified by certain characteristics thought to influence nutritional status: age, sex, social or ethnic group, environment. Each stratum is an independent universe from which samples may be drawn by one of the above-listed methods. Stratified sampling is also used where several areas or camps are to be surveyed and each of them is to be viewed separately.

The choice of sampling method depends mainly upon practical conditions. In settlements and camps, systematic random sampling is the method of choice; in a scattered population cluster sampling may have to be the choice. It must be borne in mind that in cluster sampling the sample size needs to be twice that of systematic random sampling.

SYSTEMATIC RANDOM SAMPLING

Sample size for systematic random sampling: 450 children

It is particularly recommended where the population is concentrated in an organized or structured urban setting or in a refugee camp, and where the total number of households is less than 10 000. Knowledge is required on: 1) the number of households, 2) the average number of children in the 6 months to 100 cm (5 years) group per household, 3) the total population or number of people in the universe. The recommended sample size is 450 children.

This number will ensure with a probability of 95% that the estimated prevalence will be within plus or minus 5 prevalence percent of the true prevalence irrespective of the level of prevalence. A safety margin of about 10% is included. Those wishing to include children up to 110 cm instead of 100 cm should increase the sample size to 500 children.

In practice, in camps as well as in permanent settlements, the sampling unit is the household or dwelling. Taking into account an average household size of A persons and an average proportion P of children of the right age/height in a population, the number of households needed to yield the required number of eligible children is calculated as follows:

Number of households to be visited = $450 / (A \times P)$

For example, if the average household size is 6 persons and the proportion of children under 5 years 0.15 or 15%, then 450 / (6 x 0.15) = 500 households should be visited.

If the sampling universe consists of 9000 households, the sampling interval equals 9000 / 500 = 18. Thus every 18th household is to be visited.

Further examples of calculations and procedures and more details are given in Annex 1.

Over- or underestimation of people, of households, or of the proportion of children will result in a sample that is either too small or too large. This will cause unnecessary delays and loss in precision. Estimates should therefore be as accurate as possible.

Estimates can be improved by doing a rapid count of households when planning the survey. If the number of persons in a camp or a village is known, the number of households can be estimated from a subsample of, say, 30 households; by dividing the total population of these households by 30, an average of the number of persons per household is obtained.

If the percentage of children in the appropriate 6 months to 100 cm group is overestimated, fewer households will be surveyed and the resulting sample of children will be too small. It is therefore better to underestimate than to overestimate the percentage. Information on household composition may be available from previous census data of camp or town residents.

In most developing countries, about 15% of the population will be in the required age-length group. However, in emergencies such as famines or wars this figure may be considerably lower or higher, because infants and children may have died or many adult men may be absent.

CLUSTER SAMPLING

Sample size for cluster sampling is 30 clusters of 30 children = 900 children

In cluster sampling the sample children are not spread randomly over the population but are lumped into randomly selected "clusters". It is the usual method for large populations and populations spread over a large area for which only rough estimates of the number of people are available. It may also be an advantage in large or newly established camps where numbers and ages of people are still incompletely known. However, the sample size needed to obtain the same precision is about twice that of a systematic random sample, i.e. 900 children.

This sample size ensures with a probability of 95% that the estimated prevalence will be within plus or minus 5 prevalence percent of the true prevalence, irrespective of the value of the prevalence, and assuming a correction factor of 2 (the "design effect") for cluster sampling. For reliable results it is important to examine not less than 30 clusters and not less than a total of 900 children.

For a rapid assessment in an emergency, when there is little time for preparatory work, the following sampling procedure is recommended.

The area of interest is divided on a map into sections of about equal size, following as far as possible existing geographic or administrative boundaries. Each section should have at least 300 inhabitants. A systematic sample of 30 clusters is drawn from a list of all sections and their population estimates. The total number of clusters is divided by 30 to obtain the cluster interval k starting from a randomly selected cluster on the list, every kth cluster is selected.

For example, suppose there is a total number of 183 sections. This is divided by 30 to obtain the cluster interval (183 divided by 30 = 6.1). Starting from a randomly drawn section, say section no. 15, every 6th section down the list is chosen until the 30 survey sections, the clusters, are selected. During the survey, the team starts at the centre of the cluster and chooses a direction (for example by spinning a pen on a book). The survey is started at the nearest dwelling in that direction, moving to successive houses until 30 children have been examined. At each dwelling, all eligible children should be examined.

The traditional community-based cluster sampling based on proportional sampling with a list of communities and their populations may not always be feasible in emergencies. If multiple areas or camps are to be surveyed, the most efficient approach may well be to treat each area as a stratum and to conduct systematic random sampling in each.

For another example of cluster sampling see Annex 1.

IMPORTANT CONSIDERATIONS IN SAMPLING

Every effort should be made to obtain the needed data on all children in the sample. For example, in cluster sampling all 30 children from each cluster must be seen and all eligible children in the cluster must be given equal probability of being selected.

Although random numbers are used to select sampling sites, households, and starting points, the selection procedure is never haphazard.

Samples must be selected by a rigid and defined methodology. Once the sample selection has begun, the procedure should not be changed or modified. Children must be selected for examination only by using the selected sampling procedure. Any exception will bias the estimates.

In subsequent surveys to measure changes over time, the same methodology should be used to ensure comparable results.

Only children in the households or family groups selected by the sampling procedure should be examined.

All eligible children between 6 months and 100 cm (see page 7), in each selected household or family grouping should be examined. If necessary, team members must actively search for eligible but absent children, even if a dwelling is temporarily empty, and include such children in the survey.

If a central examination site is chosen, great care must be taken to ensure that all the selected children arrive at the site. During preliminary household visits children may be numbered sequentially and the number given to the mother on a piece of paper to bring with the child to the examination site. Missing children can then be sought.

In spite of its apparently greater simplicity, in a population that is concentrated in a relatively small area, cluster sampling has no advantage over stratified or systematic sampling with its smaller sample size. Therefore, the sampling method should be carefully chosen.

For each survey the method of sample selection should be documented in writing and included in the report of survey results.

CHAPTER
5

Survey methodology

METHODS

Collect data on weight, height, sex, oedema and age

The assessment of nutritional status is based on simple anthropometric data and limited to children of preschool age, who serve to represent the general population. The data to be collected are weight, height, sex, oedema and age (if available).

The assessment is limited to protein-energy malnutrition without attempting to assess other nutritional deficiencies. No further variables should be added without considering the additional workload and delay involved.

Weight-for-height is the indicator of choice

Weight-for-height is recommended as the main or only indicator of malnutrition by most manuals and guidelines issued by UN agencies, governments, and nongovernmental organizations. It is robust, is independent of age for children, has an internationally accepted reference population, and its interpretation is based on wide experience in many parts of the world.

The indicator is formed from weight and height measurements by comparing the weight of each child to the distribution of weights of reference children of the same height. Boys and girls are treated separately, although in the field a quick analysis can be done using the table for combined sexes in Annex 2.

For each height, the weights of the reference children are distributed as an approximately normal bell-shaped curve (Figure 1), with most weights arranged around the middle of the curve, which is the mean or median of the reference weights. In order to determine the position of a measured weight in relation to the distribution of the reference weights, the distance in kg from the median of the reference curve is determined and expressed as the number of standard deviations of that distribution. This is called a standard deviation or Z-score. The standard deviation of a distribution is

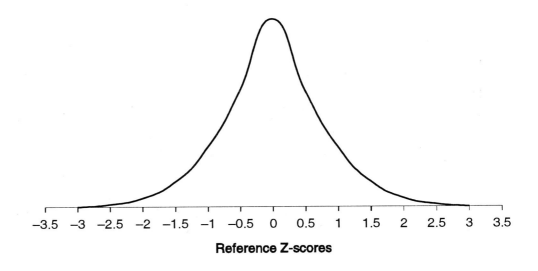

Reference Z-scores

FIGURE 1: Approximately normal weight-for-height reference curve (source: WHO)

Children with a weight-for-height of less than two standard deviations below the median are said to be below 2 standard deviations or –2 s.d. or –2 Z-scores

a measure of the width of the distribution around the mean. Standard deviation scores of children of different heights and sex are biologically equivalent and can be compared, pooled or treated statistically.

By convention, children with a weight-for-height of less than –2 s.d. or 2 Z-scores below the median of the reference are called *seriously* or *acutely malnourished*. This limit is called the cut-off point. In the normal distribution of the reference population, 2.5% of the children are below –2 s.d. by definition. There is a 1 in 43 chance that a child with weight-for-height below this point is not malnourished but is thin for other reasons. The percentage of 2.5 is considered a baseline indicating that there is no malnutrition in a population. From now, we will refer to Z-score rather than standard deviation.

A second cut-off point, –3 Z-scores (or –3 s.d.) below the median, is often used when screening malnourished children for therapeutic feeding and treatment of infections. At this cut-off there is no baseline, since at this level *all* children are *critically ill* and *severely malnourished.*

A similar approach in the past used a cut-off point of 80% of the median weight-for-height. Below this, children were considered malnourished. This method is now outdated because the 80% line does not follow the reference distribution and has different meanings at different height values. It is now replaced by the use of Z-scores. Results obtained by the two methods are not equivalent at different ages and cannot be compared or converted into each other.

Children with weight-for-height below –2 Z-scores: seriously or acutely malnourished. Below –3 Z-scores: critically, severely malnourished

It should also be noted that oedema is additional weight. Children with oedema are malnourished even though their weight may not fall below –2 Z-scores. Therefore oedema must be checked for and noted on the data sheet.

MEASURING TECHNIQUES AND RECORDING

Weight: A suitable instrument for weighing a child is a 25 kg hanging spring scale marked out in steps of 0.1 kg. After weighing pants are attached to the lower hook of the scale, the instrument is adjusted to zero. The weighing pants are then taken off and handed to the weigher. The child is freed from all heavy clothing and the weighing pants are put on. The child is then suspended from the weighing scale by the handles of the pants. It should hang freely. The weight is read to the nearest 0.1 kg with the scale at eye level. The measurer reads the value out loud, the assistant repeats it and writes it down on the recording form.

Every morning the scale should be checked against a known weight of 10 kg or less and adjusted, if necessary. If the reading is incorrect, and the scale cannot be adjusted, the springs of the scale must be changed or the scale replaced. Portable electrical scales marked in 100 g steps are also becoming available but need further testing for sturdiness under field conditions. Such a scale can be set to zero while an adult stands on it. The adult then holds the child while both are weighed, which reduces the child's distress.

Height: Children up to 2 years (23 months or 85 cm) of age are measured on a horizontal measuring board. Shoes should be removed. The child is placed gently onto the board, the soles of the feet flat against the fixed vertical part, the head near the cursor or moving part. The child should lie straight in the middle of the board, looking directly up. The assistant holds the feet firmly against the footboard and places one hand on the knees of the child, while the measurer gently holds the child's head, places the cursor against the crown of the head and reads out the length to the nearest 0.1 cm.

Children over 2 years of age (or over 85 cm) are usually measured standing on a horizontal surface against a vertical measuring device. The assistant makes sure that the child stands straight, with the heels, knees, and shoulders against the wall, while the cursor is lowered onto the crown of the head, compressing the hair. The height is read out as before, to the nearest 0.1 cm.

An easier way to measure height consists in taking the "lying down" or recumbent length of all children from 6 months to 100 cm (59 months). This method is preferred by many field workers as it avoids scaring children and making them struggle. The recumbent length is on average 0.5 cm greater than standing height. Although the difference is of no importance for the individual child, the effect on the prevalence in a population is significant, increasing the prevalence of malnutrition by 2 to 7% for prevalences between 5 and 50%. This may have to be taken into account when comparing prevalences. A correction may be made by

> **Instead of using age, which is difficult to obtain, lengths (heights) should be used to group children by approximate age: 60 to 84.9 cm for 6 months to 2 years; 85 to 100 cm for 24 to 59 months (85 to 110 cm if population not stunted)**

deducting 0.5 cm from all lengths above 84.9 cm or, if this is not possible, by correcting the calculated prevalence by using the table in Annex 4.

Age: An assessment of the ages of the children is important for two reasons: 1) malnutrition is often most marked between 6 and 18 months, which is why the age groups below and above 2 years of age should be considered separately for relief action; 2) if the height of older children is measured when they are standing, the dividing line is 2 years (see "Height" on page 21). When birth records or other documents are available, the birth date should be entered on the recording form for later computation of the exact age, or when the age is known by the mother it should be recorded in months in the appropriate space. However, in emergencies, it is often very difficult to obtain ages. *If the age is uncertain, no effort should be made to estimate it* (for example by a local calendar). Instead, lengths and heights should be used to group children by approximate age: 60 to 84.9 cm is equivalent to 6 months to 2 years, 85 to 100 cm is equivalent to 24 to 59 months (85 to 110 cm if population is not stunted).

Oedema: Oedema is the presence of abnormally large amounts of fluid in the -intercellular tissue. It is the key clinical sign of a severe form of protein-energy malnutrition carrying a very high mortality rate in young children. To diagnose oedema, moderate thumb pressure is applied to the back of the foot or the ankle for a few seconds. If there is oedema, an impression remains for some time where the oedema fluid has been pressed out of the tissue. Only if *both feet* show oedema is this recorded. Cases with oedema are separated from the rest during the analysis and are counted as severe malnutrition. A prevalence of oedema of 1 or 2% is a sign of widespread malnutrition. Children with oedema are severely ill and need immediate treatment.

Dehydration: In some circumstances recording of dehydration may be indicated. This may be important where diarrhoeal disease plays a major role and may especially affect children with evidence of wasting and weight-for-height below -2 Z-scores. The physical signs include loose skin, easy "tenting" of skin and very dry mucous membranes. These children will need immediate attention. Similarly, it may be desirable to record current diarrhoea in certain surveys.

CHAPTER 6

Data recording

In the field, findings are recorded on special data sheets, which can be either a separate form for each child or a summary form on which the data of a number of children are combined. Individual forms are useful in examination stations in camps, where children may move from station to station and heights and weights may be taken by different persons. Summary sheets are useful for mobile teams going from house to house; there is less accumulation of paper and transmission of the forms for central analysis is easier.

If computers are used for the analysis, an exact copy of the data entry screen may be printed as a field questionnaire if the *Epi-Info* software mentioned below is used. In addition to the location (district or town area, camp) the cluster number and the examination date, the form should also contain data on weight, height, sex (and age or birth date, if available), and if needed, for example for follow-up, an identification (name or number) for each child. Spaces to record the presence or absence of oedema, dehydration, and diarrhoea can also be provided.

If data analysis is to be carried out by hand in the field, forms with appropriate spaces for the results will have to be prepared. Examples of data collection forms and of a data entry screen printout are given in Figures 2 and 3. On the next page is a data collection form that can be photocopied if desired. There is room for 15 data entries on the form, so two forms would accommodate a cluster. If you make your own data collection form, it's a good idea to limit yourself to 30 entries per sheet for easier compilation.

Cluster or locality: *Camp "A"*   Date of visit: *14 May 1995*

ID	Sex m = 1 f = 2	Age months	Weight 0 0.0 kg	Height 0 0.0 cm	Oedema y = 1 n = 2	WfH > −2 Z = 0 < −2 Z = 1 < −3 Z = 2	Diarrhoea y = 1 n = 2	Dehyd y = 1 n = 2
001	2	13	07.8	71.4	2	0	1	2
002	2	17	07.9	77.5	2	1	1	2
003	1	35	11.8	85.3	2	0	2	2
004	2	.	.	.	.	.		
005	1	.	.	.				

Mean weight [   ]   Mean height [   ]   Number of children < −2 Z-scores or/and oedema [.]

FIGURE 2: *Partially filled-in summary data sheet for hand analysis*

Cluster or locality: _____ Date of visit: _____

ID	Sex m = 1 f = 2	Age months	Weight 0 0.0 kg	Height 0 0.0 cm	Oedema y = 1 n = 2	WfH > –2 Z = 0 < –2 Z = 1 < –3 Z = 2	Diarrhoea y = 1 n = 2	Dehyd y = 1 n = 2
.	.	.	.	.	.	.	.	.
.	.	.	.	.	.	.	.	.
.	.	.	.	.	.	.	.	.
.	.	.	.	.	.	.	.	.
.	.	.	.	.	.	.	.	.
.	.	.	.	.	.	.	.	.
.	.	.	.	.	.	.	.	.
.	.	.	.	.	.	.	.	.
.	.	.	.	.	.	.	.	.
.	.	.	.	.	.	.	.	.
.	.	.	.	.	.	.	.	.
.	.	.	.	.	.	.	.	.
.	.	.	.	.	.	.	.	.
.	.	.	.	.	.	.	.	.
.	.	.	.	.	.	.	.	.

Mean weight [   ]   **Mean height** [   ]   **Number of children < –2 Z-scores or/and oedema** [   ]

Source: WHO Field Guide on Rapid Nutritional Assessment in Emergencies

ANTHROPOMETRIC DATA

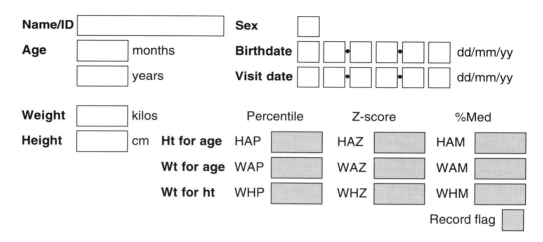

FIGURE 3: *Example of a single data sheet*
This data sheet can be obtained by printing out the Epi-Info *data screen, or you could photocopy the above. During the survey you should fill in all the boxes except for the* Ht for age, Wt for age *and* Wt for ht *boxes and the* record flag *(shaded boxes), which will be filled in automatically after you have entered the data into the computer, during data analysis.*

CHAPTER 7

Training and supervision

The quality of the survey results depends largely on adequate *training* and *supervision*.

Training includes defining the role and task of each member of a survey team, procedures to select the households, interviewing techniques, completion and coding of the survey form, and carrying out anthropometric measurements.

In general, an adequate training programme consists of three phases:

Classroom-based orientation: Demonstration of and practice in using the questionnaires and measuring heights and weights of children. All procedures should be practised by all team members.

Field practice session: Survey procedures are carried out by all team members together in an actual community to standardize procedures and organize activities, and to give team members the opportunity to practice measuring children in a survey environment. After the practice session, performances are reviewed and discussed.

Survey starting phase: In the starting phase of the actual survey, two to three teams survey together the first eight to ten households and then discuss and comment on each performance. This phase should be carried out slowly to ensure that all teams follow the same practice.

There are usually two levels of ***supervision***: the survey manager and the team leaders. The overall supervisor (team) who conducts the training and manages the overall survey may be seen as the manager(s) of the survey. In addition, each survey team should have a designated team leader who is responsible for household selection, quality of measurements, and proper completion of forms. The overall supervisor(s) needs to rotate to the different teams during the survey to monitor progress, help solving problems, and maintain comparability among the teams. Periodically, supervisors and team leaders should repeat routine measurements and record these double measurements to help maintain the quality of anthropometric techniques.

CHAPTER 8

Data analysis

ANALYSIS OF ANTHROPOMETRIC DATA

The analysis of survey results can be done in the field by hand tabulation or, if one is available, by entering the data in a portable computer (laptop or notebook computer). In either case, the weight-for-height curves of the NCHS-CDC-WHO reference are needed for the interpretation of individual weight-for-height findings. For hand tabulation, the table in Annex 2 gives the −2 Z-score weight-for-height cut-off point for the classification of malnutrition in the field.

Data analysis by hand: For the immediate decisions needed in an emergency, data analysis by hand using the table in Annex 2 will yield sufficient information. This table is for both sexes combined.

The weight of each child is checked against the −2 and −3 Z-score cut-off points given in the table in Annex 2 for the height or length measured for the individual child. If the weight is below the −2 Z-score cut-off, tick the box on the survey form as a case of malnutrition. Children with weights-for-height below −3 Z-scores are in critical condition and need immediate attention by health personnel. At the bottom of each sheet the subtotal of all cases of malnutrition including those with oedema is computed. The number of cases divided by the total number of children on the sheet and multiplied by 100 gives the prevalence for the sheet.

After the first analysis by hand the data forms must be sent to a computer facility or central survey headquarters for further analysis by computer. If local facilities are available, field data may also be entered into a computer on the spot for immediate analysis.

Data analysis by computer: For computer-based operations in the field, data processing with *Epi-Info*, *Epinut* or *Anthro* software can calculate individual weight-for-height Z-scores, which may be further analysed later.

Epi-Info software may be purchased for US$35 from USA Inc., 2075 A West Park Place, Stone Mountain, GA 30087, USA. It can be used for many types of epidemiological investigation. Since *Epi-Info* is public-domain software, it can also be copied from any existing user.

Epi-Info, *Epinut* and *Anthro* may also be obtained without cost from: Division of Nutrition (MS K25), Centers for Disease Control, Atlanta, GA 30333, USA, or from the World Health Organization, Nutrition Unit, Avenue Appia, CH-1211 Geneva 27, Switzerland, or through local WHO offices.

If the *Epi-Info* program is used for the entry of survey results, the computed Z-scores can be saved as a new variable as each record is being entered. The exact procedure is detailed in the anthropometry section of the *Epi-Info* manual. The program automatically computes weight-for-height and Z-scores, which can then be saved to the data file after checking for errors, such as extreme values. A recent version of *Epi-Info* (version 6), integrates *Epinut* into the *Epi-Info* software and has a more accessible anthropometry module than earlier versions.

Instructions on how to prepare files and enter anthropometric data for analysis are given in Annex 3. In addition, several "readme" files and help files are contained in the software itself.

In general, a weight-for-height Z-score above +4 or below –4 is likely to be an error rather than a true observation. If such values cannot be verified by remeasurement or as entry error, they should be counted as missing values. The percentage of such "likely errors" should not exceed 2% of the sample. High error values are indicative of poor measurement and/or data entry procedures. However, in extreme situations with large proportions of severely malnourished children (below –3 Z-scores) the lower limit for acceptable values may have to be dropped to a Z-score of –5.

RECOMMENDED FORMAT FOR DATA ANALYSIS

Prevalence of acute malnutrition: The prevalence of serious or acute malnutrition is the sum of the prevalence of children with weight-for-height below –2 Z-scores and the prevalence of oedema cases with weight-for-height of –2 Z-scores or more. In most cases the prevalence of oedema is only a small fraction and contributes little to the total prevalence, but in disasters with famine-like conditions the prevalence of oedema may be high and must be taken into account.

Mean Z-scores and standard deviation: The use of computer software allows the calculation of a Z-score for each child. The mean Z-score and the distribution of Z-scores of weight-for-height, i.e. the standard deviation of the Z-scores, provide useful information in addition to the prevalence below the cut-off point. The mean Z-score of a well-nourished child population should be near zero with a standard deviation of 1.0. In malnourished populations the mean Z-score will be negative, below –0.5 Z-scores. This indicates that not only has the prevalence of weight-for-height below –2 Z-scores increased, but the whole distribution has shifted to the left. A table of mean Z-scores and corresponding approximate prevalences is given in Annex 6.

The standard deviation of the weight-for-height Z-score is also important. If the standard deviation of the Z-score is significantly lower than 1.0 while the mean Z-score is significantly lower than –1.0, one may suspect that the most affected children have already died. Conversely, a high standard deviation of the weight-for-height Z-score is probably due to

A shift of the whole distribution of the population to the left underlines the fact that relief measures should be directed to the total population and not only to the fraction with a weight-for-height below –2 Z-scores

errors in the data but may produce a wrong high or low prevalence. In all cases of inconsistency between mean Z-score and prevalence, an investigation into the field situation and the survey methods is needed.

Epi-Info and other software will produce tables of frequencies for Z-score classes of 0.5 Z-score intervals and graphs of frequency distributions. A graphic representation of the difference between the distribution of the survey population and that of the reference, as in Figure 4 underlines the fact that the survey population as a whole is affected by the emergency and that relief measures should be directed at the total population rather than exclusively covering the fraction with extreme anthropometric values.

Prevalences and mean Z-scores are conveniently presented in one table. With the sample size of 450 recommended in this manual, a breakdown into two age or height groups can be made. This may reveal that a problem exists only or mainly in one of the two groups. Although dividing the sample in this fashion will lead to a loss in precision, major differences between the groups will still show. This is useful for the detection of specific causes or for targeting limited resources.

Examples of summary tables are given in Figures 5 and 6. Figure 5 could if necessary be done by hand.

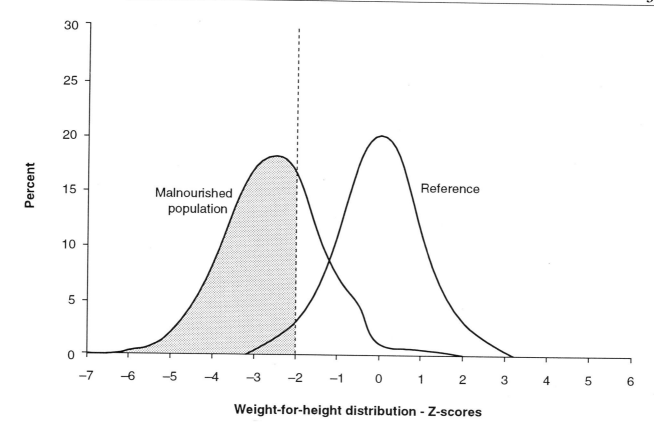

*FIGURE 4: **Major generalized downward shift of entire weight-for-height distribution** (source: WHO)*
The shaded area shows the severely malnourished (less than −2 Z-scores) portions of both reference and study populations. Note how the whole study population, even those with more than −2 Z-scores, have moved towards the lower range.

Age/length	Number of subjects	Prevalence WfH < −2 Z-scores	% with oedema
< 85 cm			
> 85 cm			
Total			

FIGURE 5: **Minimum table for hand analysis**

Age/length	Number of subjects	Prevalence WfH		Total WfH prevalence < −2 Z-scores	Mean of WfH Z-scores	s.d. of WfH Z-scores
		< −3 Z-scores	< −2 Z-scores, > −3 Z-scores			
< 24 months or < 85 cm						
> 24 months or > 85 cm						
Total						

*FIGURE 6: **More detailed table***

Source: WHO Field Guide on Rapid Nutritional Assessment in Emergencies

CHAPTER 9

Interpreting results and reporting findings

As stated in Chapter 5, in emergencies, estimates of malnutrition are based on the distribution of weight-for-height with a cut-off at -2 Z-scores. Prevalence of low weight-for-height as a direct measure of abnormal thinness in a preschool child population indicates serious health and nutritional conditions.

INTERPRETATION OF RESULTS

In order to simplify the interpretation of results and as an aid in briefing officials, the value judgements given in the table on the next page have been developed for children 6–59 months of age or 60–100 cm in length.

This classification underlines the public health importance of prevalence levels that are sometimes considered too low to require corrective action.

Percentage WfH < –2 Z-scores	Interpretation
< 5	Acceptable
5– 9.9	Poor
10–14.9	Serious
> 15	Critical

However, in the same populations much higher prevalences are often found for narrower age ranges, for example between 1 and 2 years or below 36 months.

Moreover, in already malnourished populations or in a very severe famine of some duration, much higher prevalences may be seen, which, for the purpose of setting relief priorities, might need additional classifications.

On the other hand, if prevalences are lower than could be expected from the severity of the emergency, the possibility must be considered that many children have already died.

Remember, children with a weight-for-height below –2 Z-scores are in a serious acute condition. Children with a Z-score below –3 are in a life-threatening state.

Immediate relief action can be linked to the levels of prevalence found as follows, keeping in mind the available resources:

Percentage WfH < –2 Z-scores	Relief action proposed
5– 9.9	Supplementary feeding if possible
10–14.9	Selective supplementary feeding of the malnourished is of high priority
> 15	Improve basic food supply. Additional food to all children and vulnerable groups

Long-term relief must consider the food supply of the whole family and cannot be limited to malnourished children.

REPORT OUTLINE

The report on the result of the survey should be *brief* but include all available relevant information on the overall situation.

Sections 1–3 of the report on area, type of emergency, and main changes brought about by the emergency, can be written before the survey actually takes place as they form the framework and rationale for the nutritional status survey. Sections 4–7 can be written when the survey is designed, leaving only section 8–10 to be written after the survey (refer to Chapters 8 and 9).

The following format is proposed for the report:

PROPOSED FORMAT

1. Area where the survey was held:
   - Size and geographical character
   - Population, present and before emergency
   - Administrative area
   - Character of area before the emergency (was it a food shortage area, an arid or fertile area, or in any way remarkable?)
   - Kind of population in the affected area (e.g. farmers, pastoralists, migrants)

2. Type of emergency

3. Main changes brought about by emergency:
   - Changes in food availability
   - Outbreak of diseases (which diseases)
   - Availability and functioning of health services
   - Availability of schools
   - Water and sanitation
   - Functioning of administrative infrastructure

4. Survey subjects

5. Sample sizes and sampling method

6. Number of subgroups analysed

7. Indicators and cut-off point used

8. Findings:

   - Table of prevalences and mean Z-scores, including confidence intervals and s.d. of mean Z-scores

   - Distribution curves of Z-scores comparing survey results to the reference distribution

9. Interpretation of findings

10. Conclusions and recommendations for action

Annexes

Examples of sampling

A. SYSTEMATIC SAMPLING

Example 1: A sampling interval must be computed to yield 450 children from a displaced persons' settlement with about 3000 family groupings or bush houses with an average of 1.5 children above 6 months of age and below 100 cm in length (see page 11) per grouping. For this, calculate as follows:

$$(3000 \times 1.5) / 450 = 10.0$$

In other words, every 10th family would be selected and, in each, all children who are between 6 months of age and below 100 cm in length would be measured to yield an expected sample size of 450 children. The practical implications of this sampling method are the random selection of one family grouping as the starting point and the systematic selection of every 10th family grouping counted after this starting point until the whole sampling universe is covered.

This sampling method requires initial knowledge (or good estimates) of the total population, the number of units, family groupings or bush houses, and knowledge of the average number of children in the 6 month–100 cm group per unit. It does not require the listing of each household; the households or family groupings can be counted off as the survey goes on.

Please note that, if one wishes to examine differences in the nutritional status of children in three different regions, a sample of 450 children should be taken from each region.

Example 2: Assume that a refugee camp has a total of 5000 households and a population of 40 000, about 20% of whom are children under 5 (from 6 months to 100 cm). In order to obtain a desired sample size of 450 children, first you have to determine the number of households that have to be visited to find 450 children. Thus it is estimated as follows:

1. Calculate the approximate number of children 6 months of age to 100 cm length in the camp by multiplying the total population by the estimated proportion of children of this age-length group:

$$40\ 000 \times 0.2 = 8000 \text{ children}$$

2. Divide this by the number of households in the camp to obtain the mean number of children per household:

   8000 children / 5000 households = 1.6 children per household

3. Divide the required sample size by the number of children per household to obtain the number of households to be visited (rounding up to the next integer):

   450 / 1.6 = 281.25, say 282 households should be visited.

Next, the sampling interval k is calculated by dividing the total number of households in the camp by the number of households required for the survey. Since there are 5000 households in the refugee camp and 282 are needed, the sampling interval is $5000 / 282 = 17.73$. This is rounded down to 17, which will identify $5000 / 17 = 294$ households, and these, in turn, should yield $294 \times 1.6 = 470$ children. This slightly higher number may be seen as a safeguard against possible errors in the initial estimates.

Next, a random number should be chosen between 1 and the sampling interval k, using a random-number table or other source, such as the end digits of a currency note. The survey team picks a starting point, which may be a corner of the camp or town, if the site is well organized (the team will move up and down rows of houses), or it may choose the centre as a starting point, if the houses are irregularly arranged (the team will move in a circular fashion). From the starting point, the team counts the houses until the chosen random number is reached and starts the first examination. After the first house, every kth (17th) house is visited until the needed sample is obtained.

The sampling interval is 20. A random number of 12 is picked from a currency note. The survey team begins in the northwest corner of the camp, counts out the first 12 households, and visits the 12th household where there is one child under 5, who is examined. They then continue eastwards, counting the households as they go, until they have passed another 20 households to house no. 32. This house contains 2 children, who are included in the survey. They continue counting until they reach the end of the first row and double-back westward into the second row. When the 20th household is reached (household no. 52), they include it in the survey. There are no children in this household, so they proceed 20 households further on, to household no. 72. They continue sampling every 20th household (nos. 92, 112, 132, etc.) until they reach the southeast corner of the camp.

B. CLUSTER SAMPLING

In addition to the example given in Chapter 4, a somewhat more elaborate approach is given below.

While, with random and stratified sampling, all camps or villages of interest are included in the universe from which the sample is drawn, in a cluster sampling survey, a first sample is chosen from such units.

The first step in the sampling process is to obtain the best available census data for each city, village, or camp in the area of interest. In most circumstances, the total population rather than the population of children under 5 is used to develop the sampling frame, since children form a relatively stable fraction of the population and the total population figures are usually easier to obtain.

In a stable population, such as a drought-affected region with little in- and out-migration, a census that may be several years old may still be acceptable as a base for population proportionate sampling. However, in refugee situations where influx continues, reliable up-to-date counts are important for a valid sample.

Next, a list with three columns should be made. The first column should include the name of each geographic unit (e.g. village, town, or district). The second column should contain the population of each unit. The third column should contain the cumulative population (adding the population of each unit to the combined population figure of the preceding units). The list can reflect the order given in the national census or may be arranged from largest to smallest to assure good representation.

The sampling interval is obtained by dividing the total population by the desired number of clusters, which is usually 30. A random number is chosen, for example from a bank note, as the starting point, and the sampling interval is added sequentially to the random number until 30 numbers are chosen. Each number chosen represents the population of a geographic unit.

The corresponding sites in the first column of the list are the cluster sites. The 30 clusters should be plotted on a map of the area and divided among the survey teams.

When a survey team reaches a cluster, it moves towards the centre of the cluster, a direction is chosen (e.g. by spinning a pen on a book), and the survey is started at the nearest dwelling in that direction, moving to successive houses until 30 children have been examined. Efforts must be made to locate and examine temporarily absent children.

ANNEX 2

CDC/WHO normalized reference table of weight-for-height (length)

TABLE 1. **CDC/WHO normalized reference weight for height and length (combined sexes) 58.0 to 110 cm**

Length* cm	Weight kg −2 Z-score	−3 Z-score	Length* cm	Weight kg −2 Z-score	−3 Z-score
58.0	3.9	3.3	71.5	7.3	6.5
58.5	4.0	3.4	72.0	7.4	6.6
59.0	4.1	3.5	72.5	7.6	6.7
59.5	4.2	3.6	73.0	7.7	6.8
60.0	4.4	3.7	73.5	7.8	6.9
60.5	4.5	3.8	74.0	7.9	7.0
61.0	4.6	4.0	74.5	8.0	7.1
61.5	4.8	4.1	75.0	8.1	7.2
62.0	4.9	4.2	75.5	8.2	7.3
62.5	5.0	4.3	76.0	8.3	7.4
63.0	5.1	4.4	76.5	8.4	7.5
63.5	5.3	4.6	77.0	8.5	7.6
64.0	5.4	4.7	77.5	8.6	7.7
64.5	5.5	4.8	78.0	8.7	7.8
65.0	5.6	4.9	78.5	8.8	7.9
65.5	5.8	5.0	79.0	8.9	8.0
66.0	5.9	5.2	79.5	8.9	8.1
66.5	6.0	5.3	80.0	9.0	8.2
67.0	6.1	5.4	80.5	9.1	8.2
67.5	6.3	5.6	81.0	9.2	8.3
68.0	6.4	5.7	81.5	9.3	8.4
68.5	6.5	5.8	82.0	9.4	8.5
69.0	6.7	5.9	82.5	9.5	8.6
69.5	6.8	6.1	83.0	9.6	8.7
70.0	6.9	6.2	83.5	9.7	8.8
70.5	7.0	6.3	84.0	9.8	8.9
71.0	7.2	6.4	84.5	9.8	8.9

*Length below 85 cm; height from 85 cm, or 2 years and above. If you use this table with children above 85 cm who were measured *lying down* you must correct the prevalence (see page 21 and Annex 4)

Continued . . .

TABLE 1. **CDC/WHO normalized reference weight for height and length (combined sexes) 58.0 to 110 cm** *Continued*

Height* cm	Weight *kg* -2 Z-score	-3 Z-score	Height* cm	Weight *kg* -2 Z-score	-3 Z-score
85.0	9.8	8.8	98.5	12.5	11.2
85.5	9.9	8.8	99.0	12.6	11.3
86.0	10.0	8.9	99.5	12.7	11.4
86.5	10.1	9.0	100.0	12.9	11.5
87.0	10.2	9.1	100.5	13.0	11.6
87.5	10.3	9.2	101.0	13.1	11.7
88.0	10.4	9.3	101.5	13.2	11.8
88.5	10.5	9.4	102.0	13.3	11.9
89.0	10.6	9.5	102.5	13.4	12.0
89.5	10.7	9.6	103.0	13.5	12.1
90.0	10.8	9.7	103.5	13.6	12.2
90.5	10.9	9.8	104.0	13.7	12.3
91.0	11.0	9.8	104.5	13.9	12.4
91.5	11.1	9.9	105.0	14.0	12.5
92.0	11.2	10.0	105.5	14.1	12.6
92.5	11.3	10.1	106.0	14.2	12.7
93.0	11.4	10.2	106.5	14.3	12.8
93.5	11.5	10.3	107.0	14.5	12.9
94.0	11.6	10.4	107.5	14.6	13.0
94.5	11.7	10.5	108.0	14.7	13.2
95.0	11.8	10.6	108.5	14.8	13.2
95.5	11.9	10.7	109.0	15.0	13.4
96.0	12.0	10.8	109.5	15.1	13.5
96.5	12.1	10.9	110.0	15.2	13.6
97.0	12.2	10.9			
97.5	12.3	11.0			
98.0	12.4	11.1			

*Length below 85 cm; height from 85 cm, or 2 years and above. If you use this table with children above 85 cm who were measured *lying down* you must correct the prevalence (see page 21 and Annex 4)

ANNEX 3

Guidelines for using *Epi-Info*

HOW TO CARRY OUT DATA ANALYSIS USING EPI-INFO *VERSION 5*

To be able to follow the instructions you must have *Epi-Info* version 5 already installed on your computer's hard disk.

If that has not yet been done, do so first, using the instructions provided with the diskettes.

Now perform the following steps:

1. Go to the DOS-prompt and type `cd c:\epi5` or, if you are already working in *Epi-Info*, choose `Quit Epi-Info` from the `Epi-Info` menu screen.

2. After any of the steps above, your screen now should show the following prompt: `c:\epi5`

3. You now have to decide on a name for your datafile. For the sake of this example we have chosen to call our data file EMRO. When you perform this operation yourself, you can use any other name, or you can also of course use the name EMRO.

Please note that for each separate dataset you need to make a separate datafile using the steps below.

You are now going to make all the necessary files to support your data analysis. To do that, you will copy a number of important files.

Just type at the prompt:

`copy europe.* emro.*` Then press the Enter key.

You will see a note that four files have been copied and the prompt returns.

Remember that this example uses `emro` as name for the new data file. You can use any name of your choosing. Just replace the word `emro` by the name of your choice in all the steps described.

4. Type `epi` and from the `Epi-Info` menu choose EPED.

    You do this by highlighting the bar called EPED and pressing Enter or by choosing the letter highlighted in the word EPED.

5. Press F2 (file). You now see a menu on which the sentence `open file this window` is highlighted. Press Enter. You will see a box prompting you to type in the file you want to open. Type `emro.bat`.

6. On your screen you have a short list of sentences. In the third line, change the words ENTER EUROPE to ENTER EMRO.

7. Press F9 (save) and F10 (done).

It is important to note that if this step was not carried out successfully the analysis cannot be carried out. Therefore repeat step 5 and make sure the text in line 3 reads ENTER EMRO. Then press F10 and continue.

8. From the Epi-Info menu choose Quit Epi-Info.

9. At the c:\epi5> prompt, type emro. You will now see the questionnaire on screen.

10. Follow instructions and enter the data for each child separately. Make sure you enter the figures correctly. If you have no record of ages, skip the boxes for age and visit date.

   After checking that the record has been properly entered press y[es] to save the record, or n[o] if you need to correct it.

   Continue till you have entered all the children. You have now completed the data entry. Now press F10 (done).

   You will automatically have returned to the prompt.

   Type epi.

   From the Epi-Info menu now choose Analysis.

   When the analysis screen appears type read emro.

   You can then proceed with the analysis of your data, using the commands under F2 and the help under F1, as well as the manual provided with the software.

Please note that, for those who wish to make alterations to the data-entry screen, i.e. the questionnaire, the following remarks apply:

- The questionnaire file (EMRO.QES) can be modified to meet your special requirements. You can add variables or use ID instead of NAME. To do this you only need to specify the type of variable fields, i.e. text versus numeric versus yes/no, etc. To avoid complications, it is best to add new variables before the WEIGHT and HEIGHT variables in the QES file.

- To reduce data entry errors, edit limits can be included by modifying the EMRO.CHK file. This file can be accessed by selecting the **CHECK** option from the main menu, after which the instructions on the screen will guide you through.

- The *Epi-Info* manual and "readme" files are helpful in guiding the user in this process.

Correction for prevalences for children above 85 cm who were measured lying down

In groups of children, the measured supine length is on average 0.5 cm larger than the measured height. If children above 2 years or above 85 cm are measured lying down instead of standing up, the influence on the calculated prevalence may be of practical importance. For example, if a boy measures 86.5 cm lying down, the computer subroutine uses the reference weight distribution for boys of 86.5 cm instead of the correct 86.0 cm. Since the median weight of the reference at 86.0 cm is 0.2 kg below that at 86.5 cm, the cut-off at −2 s.d. for 85.6 is too far out and the calculated prevalence would be too large. This error increases with the prevalence. Using a reference s.d. of 1.1 kg, a correction for different prevalences has been developed which may be subtracted from the calculated prevalence. Although the relation is curvilinear, a linear function seemed adequate for a range from 5 to 50% prevalence, and a linear regression equation was set up for the correction factor y:

$$y = 2.2 + 0.1x$$

x being the apparent prevalence from which *y* has to be deducted. Values for different prevalences are given in the table below.

This correction may be applied if the difference is of practical importance.

Prevalence in percent (x)	to be deducted (y)
5	2.7
10	3.2
20	4.2
30	5.2
40	6.2
50	7.2

Source: W. Keller

Estimation of low weight-for-height from mean weight and mean height

In an emergency, the transmittal of anthropometric measurements to a central station for analysis and utilization may be hindered by impairments in communications. A simplified method was devised to estimate the prevalence of malnutrition from summary data that are easily reported even by radio telephone.

The estimate is based on the observation that in a malnourished population the distribution of weight-for-height Z-scores is usually shifted to the left without any major change in the width of the distribution. The proportion of children below the cut-off point at −2 Z-scores may be estimated from the observed mean weight for the mean height and the weight for this height in the reference population and by estimating the standard deviation of the reference weight at the mean height for the unknown distribution (i.e. the sample). If the cut-off point is set at 2 s.d.

(or Z-scores) below the reference median, the calculation follows the equation:

$$Z = (M - m) / S$$

where m is the observed mean weight, M is the reference median weight for the observed mean height, and S the standard deviation of the same reference weight. M and S can be found in Table 1. The tail size or prevalence corresponding to the resulting Z value is given in Table 2.

TABLE 1. **Reference median weight for observed height and standard deviation(s)**

Mean height cm	Weight for height kg	s.d. kg	Mean height cm	Weight for height kg	s.d. kg
80	10.9	0.87	90	13.3	1.17
81	11.1	0.87	91	13.5	1.2
82	11.3	0.87	92	13.7	1.2
83	11.5	0.9	93	14.0	1.23
84	11.7	0.9	94	14.2	1.23
85	12.1	1.06	95	14.5	1.27
86	12.3	1.1	96	14.7	1.27
87	12.6	1.13	97	15.0	1.33
88	12.8	1.13	98	15.2	1.33
89	13.0	1.13	99	15.5	1.37
			100	15.7	1.37

TABLE 2. **Tail of distribution for different Z**

Z	Percentage	Z	Percentage
0.1	2.9	1.1	18
0.2	3.6	1.2	21
0.3	4.5	1.3	24
0.4	5.5	1.4	27
0.5	7	1.5	31
0.6	8	1.6	34
0.7	10	1.7	38
0.8	12	1.8	42
0.9	14	1.9	46
1.0	16	2.0	50

Source: W. Keller, EMRO, and Jenny Allan, SCF (UK)

The procedure is illustrated by the following example based on three studies among groups of displaced.

Item	Group 1	Group 2	Group 3
No. of cases	3900	1799	2396
Mean weight m (kg)	10.89	10.78	11.85
Mean height	85.92	86.24	89.64
Reference weight for mean height M (kg)	12.3	12.4	13.1
Reference s.d. at mean height (kg)	1.10	1.12	1.13
$M - m$ (kg)	1.4	1.6	1.3
$(M - m) / S$	1.272	1.428	1.150
Estimated prevalence (%)	23.3	28.8	19.8
Prevalence from computer analysis (%)	23.4	27.3	19.4

Mean Z-scores and corresponding prevalences below –2 Z-scores

Mean Z-score	Prevalence < –2 Z-scores	Mean Z-score	Prevalence < –2 Z-scores
–3.0	84	–1.0	16
–2.5	69	–0.9	14
–2.4	66	–0.8	12
–2.3	62	–0.7	10
–2.2	58	–0.6	8
–2.1	54	–0.5	6.7
–2.0	50	–0.4	6.0
–1.9	46	–0.3	4.5
–1.8	42	–0.2	3.6
–1.7	38	–0.1	2.8
–1.6	34	0	2.3
–1.5	31	+0.1	1.8
–1.4	27	+0.2	1.4
–1.3	24	+0.3	1.1
–1.2	21	+0.4	0.8
–1.1	18	+0.5	0.6

Equipment needed

- Length board
- Unstretchable measuring tapes
- Weighing scale, 25 kg x 100 g (hanging scale) or electronic weighing scale with zeroing capacity
- Rope, extra weighing pants
- Standard weight (10 kg) or water container with known filled weight
- Questionnaires, data sheets
- Pencils, erasers, sharpeners, drawing pins
- Clipboards, staplers, sticky tape, rubber bands
- Tables, pocket calculator and/or notebook computer
- This field guide

SOME SUPPLIERS OF WEIGHING AND MEASURING EQUIPMENT

A Fleischhaeker, G - Postfach 1249, 58207 Schwerte/Ruhr, Germany

Medical Export Group of the Netherlands BV, P.O. 598, 4200 AN Gorinchem, the Netherlands

Rowen Equipment Ltd, Unit 4, Ford Farm Industrial Complex, Braintree Road, Dunmow, Essex CM6 1HU, UK

ANNEX 8

Further reading

- The Management of Nutritional Emergencies in Large Populations (revised edition) WHO 1995 (in press)

- Sample Size Determination in Health Studies—A Practice Manual S.K. Lwanga and S. Lemeshow, WHO, Geneva, 1991

- Measuring Change in Nutritional Status, WHO, Geneva, 1983

- An Evaluation of Infant Growth, Nutrition Unit, WHO, Geneva, 1994

- Physical Status: the Use and Interpretation of Anthropometry—Report of an Expert committee, WHO, Geneva, 1995 (in press).